Compassion in Crisis:

The Balancing Act of a Caregiver

TABLE OF CONTENTS

Chapter I. Introduction

My Personal Journey as a Caregiver

Why Compassionate Care Matters

Challenges Faced by Individuals with Cancer, Heart Conditions and Mental Illness

Providing Support: The Importance of Empathy and Understanding

Chapter II

Understanding Cancer Through My Eyes

My Experience with Supporting Loved Ones Facing Cancer

Insights into Different Types of Cancer and Their Impact on Individuals

Navigating Treatments and Managing Side Effects

Emotional and Psychological Support: Sharing My Strategies for Being There in Times of Need

Chapter III

Chapter IV

Chapter V

Compassion in Crisis: The Balancing Act of a Caregiver

CHAPTER I. INTRODUCTION

My Personal Journey as a Caregiver

My personal journey as a caregiver has been a profound and multifaceted experience, shaped by the challenges of simultaneously caring for my mother, who battles dementia, my niece who is fighting cancer, and my sister who struggles with mental illness. Each day presents a new set of obstacles, emotions, and triumphs as I navigate the complexities of providing care and support to my loved ones in their time of need.

Caring for my mother, who is grappling with dementia, has been a journey marked by both heartache and moments of profound connection. Witnessing the gradual decline of her cognitive abilities has been incredibly difficult, yet amidst the challenges, there are glimpses of the vibrant woman she once was. As her caregiver, I strive to preserve her dignity and quality of life while embracing the role of companion and advocate in her journey through dementia.

In addition to caring for my mother, I am also supporting my niece through her battle with cancer. The weight of her diagnosis hangs heavy in the air, yet amidst the fear and uncertainty, there is an unwavering spirit of resilience and hope. As her caregiver, I am committed to providing her with the love, strength, and support she needs to navigate the challenges of cancer treatment and emerge victorious in her fight against the disease.

It takes careful balancing to meet the needs of caring for my mother and niece while also helping my sister with her mental health issues. Even though there are times when I feel like my obligations are too much to manage, I find strength in my wife and the love and bond that unite our family. We journey through life's highs and lows together, comforting one another with the love and support that binds us together even in the most difficult circumstances.

Providing care for family members dealing with a wide range of health issues has imparted priceless knowledge on empathy, compassion, and the human spirit's tenacity. Additionally, it has made me more aware of how fleeting life is and how crucial it is to treasure every second we have together. We have united as a family in the face of hardship, leaning on one another for support and finding hope when all else seemed lost.

Being a caregiver has brought me both joy and sadness, but no matter what, I am thankful for the chance to support my loved ones during their tough times. I am motivated by the conviction that, working together, we can conquer any challenge and come out stronger and more resilient than before, even though the road ahead may be long and difficult. My experience as a caregiver serves as a tribute to the strength of love, compassion, and unwavering loyalty in the face of hardship.

WHY COMPASSIONATE CARE MATTERS

Compassionate care is paramount when fulfilling the role of caregiver to loved ones facing health challenges such as dementia and mental illness. As a caregiver to my mother, who battles dementia, and my sister, who struggles with mental illness, I have witnessed firsthand the transformative power of compassion in providing support and comfort during their time of need.

Primarily, compassionate care acknowledges the inherent dignity and worth of the individual, regardless of their health condition. For my mother, who grapples with the cognitive decline of dementia, and my sister, who navigates the complexities of mental illness, compassionate care affirms their humanity and honors their unique experiences, fears, and emotions.

A sense of understanding and connection between the caregiver and the recipient is another benefit of caring for someone with sympathy. As a caregiver, I try to develop empathy and attentive listening skills to comprehend the needs and viewpoints of my mother and sister. Compassionate care creates a safe and supportive environment where my loved ones feel heard, valued, and respected by encouraging open communication and genuine empathy.

By attending to the patient's emotional, psychological, and spiritual needs in addition to the physical symptoms of their illness, thoughtful treatment fosters holistic well-being. Compassionate care for my mother and sister involves offering companionship, emotional support, and opportunities for meaningful engagement and connection. This is because they are dealing with both mental illness and dementia.

Self-care is important for both the caregiver and the recipient, and compassionate care acknowledges this. To prioritize my own well-being while managing the responsibilities of caregiving, I engage in self-compassion exercises, ask for help when I need it, and take breaks when necessary. I can give my mother and sister more compassionate care when I put self-care first because I can be patient, empathetic, and resilient for them.

Moreover, compassionate care extends beyond the realm of physical tasks and medical treatments to encompass advocacy and empowerment. As a caregiver, I advocate for my mother's and sister's needs and rights, ensuring that they receive the best possible care and support. By advocating for their well-being, I empower them to navigate the challenges of their illnesses with dignity, autonomy, and agency.

A caring attitude also promotes optimism as well as perseverance in the face of hardship. My mother and sister find comfort and strength in the kindness and support they receive from their caregivers and loved ones, despite the difficulties posed by dementia and mental illness. We develop a sense of toughness and expectation that gets us through even the worst of times by fostering a culture of understanding and kindness.

When providing care for loved ones dealing with health issues like dementia and mental illness, caring compassion is crucial. Compassionate care makes sure that my mother and sister get the support and comfort they need to handle the complexities of their illnesses with grace and dignity. It does this by recognizing the inherent dignity of the individual, fostering connection, and understanding, promoting holistic well-being, emphasizing self-care, advocating for needs and rights, and fostering spirit and hope.

CHALLENGES FACED BY INDIVIDUALS WITH CANCER, HEART CONDITIONS, AND MENTAL ILLNESS

Individuals facing cancer, heart conditions, and mental illness confront a myriad of challenges that deeply impact their lives physically, emotionally, and psychologically. These challenges vary in nature and severity but collectively pose significant hurdles that can profoundly affect the quality of life for those affected.

For those battling cancer, the challenges are multifaceted. The physical toll of the disease and its treatments, such as chemotherapy, radiation therapy, and surgery, often leads to debilitating side effects such as fatigue, nausea, pain, and hair loss. Additionally, the emotional burden of facing a life-threatening illness and the uncertainty of the future can be overwhelming. Coping with the financial strain of medical bills and navigating the complex healthcare system further exacerbates the challenges faced by individuals with cancer.

Heart conditions present a unique set of challenges characterized by the potential for sudden and life-threatening events such as heart attacks, strokes, and cardiac arrest. Individuals with heart conditions may struggle with managing symptoms such as chest pain, shortness of breath, and fatigue, which can severely impact their ability to perform daily activities and maintain an excellent quality of life. Lifestyle changes, including dietary modifications, exercise regimens, and medication adherence, are often necessary to manage heart conditions effectively. Furthermore, the fear and anxiety associated with living with a chronic and potentially life-threatening illness can take a significant toll on mental health and well-being.

Mental illness presents its own set of challenges that are often invisible yet deeply impactful. Conditions such as depression, anxiety, bipolar disorder, and schizophrenia can significantly impair an individual's ability to function in various aspects of life, including work, relationships, and daily activities. Stigma and discrimination surrounding mental illness can exacerbate feelings of shame, isolation, and hopelessness, making it challenging for individuals to seek help and access appropriate treatment. Moreover, navigating the mental healthcare system and finding effective treatment options can be daunting and overwhelming for both individuals and their families.

Beyond the physical and emotional challenges, individuals facing cancer, heart conditions, and mental illness often grapple with social and interpersonal difficulties. Maintaining relationships with family, friends, and coworkers may become strained as individuals cope with the demands of their illnesses. Feelings of guilt, shame, and self-doubt may arise, further complicating social interactions and exacerbating feelings of isolation and loneliness. Moreover, the loss of independence and autonomy that often accompanies chronic illness can lead to feelings of frustration, anger, and grief.

Access to comprehensive and affordable healthcare is another significant challenge faced by individuals with cancer, heart conditions, and mental illness. Disparities in healthcare access and quality can exacerbate existing health inequalities, particularly for marginalized and underserved populations. Limited access to healthcare services, including preventive care, diagnostic testing, and specialty treatments, can impede individuals' ability to manage their illnesses effectively and achieve optimal health outcomes.

The journey of living with cancer, heart conditions, or mental illness is fraught with challenges that test the resilience, courage, and strength of individuals and their families. Despite the many obstacles they face, individuals affected by these illnesses demonstrate remarkable strength and perseverance in their quest for health, well-being, and quality of life. By raising awareness, advocating for equitable access to healthcare, and providing compassionate support, we can work together to alleviate the burdens faced by individuals with cancer, heart conditions, and mental illness and foster a more inclusive and supportive society for all.

PROVIDING SUPPORT: THE IMPORTANCE OF EMPATHY AND UNDERSTANDING

The first step in providing support is to develop feelings of care and compassion for the people we look after. Effective caregiving is based on empathy because it enables us to put ourselves in our loved ones' shoes and view the world from their point of view. By sharing our understanding of their problems, feelings, and experiences, we build the connection and trust that are necessary to offer genuine support.

Fostering compassion and understanding for the people we look after is the first step in offering support. As it enables us to put ourselves in our loved ones' shoes and view the world from their perspective, empathy is the cornerstone of providing effective care. We build the trust and connection necessary to offer genuine support by becoming emotionally and psychologically attuned to their experiences, struggles, and feelings.

Apart from that, establishing a compassionate and understanding atmosphere facilitates the dismantling of barriers and lessens feelings of loneliness. Those who struggle with illnesses like mental illness, heart problems, or cancer frequently feel stigmatized or misunderstood by society. They can express themselves freely and without fear of repercussions in the safe and encouraging environment we provide by showing them empathy and understanding.

Empathy and understanding enable us to provide more effective and holistic care to our loved ones. By recognizing the emotional, psychological, and spiritual dimensions of their health challenges, we can offer support that addresses their whole being, not just their physical symptoms. This may include providing emotional support, assisting with practical tasks, advocating for their needs, and facilitating access to resources and services that promote their well-being.

Stronger ties between family members and those receiving care are also fostered by empathy and understanding. People trust their caregivers more and rely on their loved ones for support when they feel heard, validated, and supported. As they travel through their shared health journey, this feeling of unity and support can be a source of resiliency and strength for both the care recipient and the caregiver.

In the end, it is impossible to overestimate the significance of empathy and understanding in creating the conditions necessary for offering support. We can create a supportive and empowering environment that promotes healing, resilience, and well-being by learning to empathize with and understand our loved ones who are dealing with health challenges. It is our duty as caregivers to guide with feelings of sympathy and empathy, appreciating the intrinsic value and dignity of every person we look after and enabling them to live life to the fullest despite any health issues.

CHAPTER II
Understanding Cancer Through My Eyes

It has been an incredibly personal journey for me to understand cancer, and it has changed the way I view resilience, love, and life in general. Having been a caregiver for loved ones dealing with this powerful enemy, I have had a close-up view of the difficulties and complexities involved in negotiating the maze of cancer diagnosis, treatment, and recovery. In addition to broadening my empathy and comprehension, my experiences have also made me more aware of the incredible bravery and strength that each person battling this illness possesses.

My journey with cancer began with the diagnosis of a dear family member, and from that moment onward, my world was forever altered. The initial shock and disbelief gave way to a relentless determination to support my loved one through every step of their journey.

As I accompanied them to doctor's appointments, sat by their side during chemotherapy sessions, and held their hand through moments of fear and uncertainty, I gained invaluable insights into the physical, emotional, and psychological toll that cancer exacts on those it touches.

Witnessing the transformative power of resilience and hope in the face of cancer has been both humbling and awe-inspiring. Despite the ravages of the disease and the grueling nature of treatment, I have seen firsthand the indomitable spirit of individuals who refuse to be defined by their diagnosis. Their unwavering courage, optimism, and determination to fight against all odds have left an indelible imprint on my heart and soul, reminding me of the boundless capacity of the human spirit to triumph over adversity.

My understanding of cancer has also increased my appreciation of the value of compassionate care and all-encompassing support. I now understand the importance of attending to the emotional, psychological, and spiritual needs of cancer patients in addition to their medical interventions and treatments. It is impossible to overestimate the role that human connection plays in easing the effects of cancer, whether it takes the form of lending a sympathetic ear, giving consoling support, or just being a source of inspiration and strength.

My experience with cancer has brought to light the critical role that empowerment and advocacy play in ensuring that people receive the support and care they are entitled to. Being a voice for those affected by cancer is crucial in fostering positive outcomes and promoting dignity and autonomy. I have learned this from navigating the complexity of the healthcare system to advocating for access to quality treatment and support services.

Recognizing cancer through my eyes has been a transformative and enlightening experience that has deepened my empathy, strengthened my resolve, and reaffirmed my commitment to supporting those affected by this disease. As I continue this journey, I am reminded of the importance of compassion, resilience, and hope in navigating the challenges of cancer and emerging stronger and more united in our shared fight against this formidable adversary.

MY EXPERIENCE WITH SUPPORTING LOVED ONES FACING CANCER

Supporting loved ones with cancer has been a challenging yet rewarding journey for me. The moment I found out that a family member or friend had been diagnosed with cancer, my world turned upside down. The initial shock and fear were overwhelming, but I knew that I had to be there for them every step of the way. From accompanying them to doctor's appointments to providing emotional support and practical assistance, I have been committed to supporting my loved ones through their cancer journey.

One of the most important ways I have supported my loved ones with cancer is by being a constant source of emotional support. Cancer can be a lonely and isolating experience, and having someone to listen, comfort, and reassure them has been crucial for my loved ones. I make sure to check in regularly, offer a shoulder to lean on, and provide a listening ear whenever they need to talk about their fears, concerns, or hopes.

I found myself taking on various roles and responsibilities to support my loved one through their cancer treatment. From accompanying them to medical appointments and treatment sessions to helping manage medications, appointments, and coordination, I became their advocate, confidant, and caretaker all rolled into one. It was a role that demanded flexibility, empathy, and resilience, but it was also one filled with moments of deep connection and shared strength.

In addition to emotional support, I have also been actively involved in helping my loved ones navigate the complex healthcare system. This includes researching treatment options, scheduling appointments, coordinating care with their medical team, and advocating for their needs. I have made it a priority to stay informed about their medical condition and treatment plan so that I can be a knowledgeable and effective advocate on their behalf.

Another way I have supported my loved ones with cancer is by helping them with practical tasks and daily activities. This can range from preparing meals and running errands to managing household chores and providing transportation to and from medical appointments. By taking on these responsibilities, I have been able to alleviate some of the stress and burden on my loved ones, allowing them to focus on their healing and recovery.

I have also supported my loved ones with cancer by attending doctor's appointments and treatment sessions with them. This has been a valuable opportunity to ask questions, seek clarification, and ensure that my loved ones receive the best care possible. By being present at these appointments, I have been able to offer my support, lend a listening ear, and provide a sense of comfort and reassurance during what can be a stressful and overwhelming time.

I have been actively involved in researching and learning about their specific type of cancer, treatment options, and potential side effects. By educating myself on these topics, I have been better equipped to provide informed support and guidance to my loved ones. I have also connected with other caregivers and support groups to learn from their experiences and gather valuable insights on how to best support my loved ones through their cancer journey.

I have made it a priority to respect and honor my loved ones' autonomy and decision-making abilities throughout their cancer treatment. While I offer my support and guidance, I also recognize that my loved ones have the right to make decisions about their care that are in line with their values and preferences. I have encouraged open communication and dialogue, creating a safe space for my loved ones to express their needs and concerns.

I have supported my loved ones with cancer by fostering a sense of hope and positivity. Cancer can often feel like a dark and overwhelming cloud, but I have made it a point to remind my loved ones of the strength, resilience, and courage they possess. I have celebrated their victories, no matter how small, and offered words of encouragement and inspiration to keep their spirits lifted during challenging times.

Another important aspect of supporting my loved ones with cancer has been advocating for their needs and ensuring that their voices are heard within the healthcare system. I have been a strong and vocal advocate, speaking up on behalf of my loved ones to ensure that they receive the best possible care and support. I have collaborated closely with their medical team to address any concerns or challenges, advocating for personalized and compassionate care that meets their unique needs.

I have supported my loved ones by creating a sense of normalcy and routine in their daily lives. Cancer can disrupt one's sense of stability and control, so I have tried to maintain routines, engage in activities they enjoy, and provide a sense of normalcy amidst the chaos. By creating a sense of predictability and comfort, I have helped my loved ones feel more grounded and supported during their cancer journey.

I have supported my loved ones with cancer by being a source of strength and resilience in the face of adversity. I have remained positive, hopeful, and steadfast in my support, even during the most challenging moments. By being a consistent and unwavering presence in their lives, I have helped my loved ones feel supported, empowered, and uplifted as they navigate their cancer journey.

While supporting loved ones with cancer has been a profound and transformative experience for me. By offering emotional support, navigating the healthcare system, assisting with practical tasks, attending appointments, educating myself on their condition, respecting their autonomy, fostering hope and positivity, advocating for their needs, maintaining routines, and being a source of strength and resilience, I have been able to provide the unwavering support that my loved ones need during their cancer journey. It is a privilege to walk alongside them, offer my support, and be a source of comfort and encouragement as they face the challenges of cancer with grace and resilience.

INSIGHTS INTO DIFFERENT TYPES OF CANCER & THEIR IMPACT ON INDIVIDUALS

I have personally witnessed the devastating impact that several types of cancer can have on individuals. It is a topic that hits close to home for me, as I have seen loved ones battle this disease. Cancer is not just a physical ailment; it affects every aspect of a person's life - their physical health, emotional well-being, and even their relationships.

One of the most common types of cancer is breast cancer. As a woman, the thought of being diagnosed with breast cancer is terrifying. It can lead to feelings of fear, sadness, and uncertainty about the future. The impact of breast cancer goes beyond the physical pain and discomfort of treatments like chemotherapy and radiation. It can also affect a person's self-esteem and body image, as surgeries like mastectomy may be necessary.

Another type of cancer that has a profound impact on individuals is lung cancer. This disease is often associated with smoking, but it can affect non-smokers as well. The impact of lung cancer is not limited to physical symptoms such as coughing, shortness of breath, and chest pain. It can also lead to feelings of guilt and shame, as society often stigmatizes lung cancer patients due to the association with smoking.

Leukemia, a cancer of the blood and bone marrow, is yet another type of cancer that has a significant impact on individuals. The impact of leukemia is not only felt by the person diagnosed but also by their loved ones. The emotional toll of watching a loved one go through grueling treatments and the uncertainty of the outcome can be overwhelming. It can strain relationships and cause immense stress for everyone involved.

Prostate cancer, primarily affecting men, is another type of cancer that has a profound impact on individuals. The impact of prostate cancer goes beyond the physical symptoms such as difficulty urinating and erectile dysfunction. It can also lead to feelings of emasculation and a loss of identity for men. Treatments for prostate cancer, such as surgery and radiation, can have long-lasting effects on a person's quality of life.

Skin cancer, including melanoma, is a type of cancer that often goes unnoticed until it reaches an advanced stage. The impact of skin cancer is not just physical; it can also have a significant emotional impact. The fear of recurrence and the constant need for vigilant sun protection can take a toll on a person's mental well-being.

Pancreatic cancer is one of the most aggressive and deadliest forms of cancer. The impact of pancreatic cancer is devastating, both physically and emotionally. The survival rate for pancreatic cancer is low, and the treatments can be harsh and debilitating. It can cause severe pain, weight loss, and digestive issues, making it incredibly challenging for individuals to maintain their quality of life.

Several types of cancer have a profound impact on individuals. The physical, emotional, and psychological toll of this disease cannot be underestimated. It is crucial to support and empathize with those affected by cancer and to continue working towards finding better treatments and a cure.

NAVIGATING TREATMENTS & MANAGING SIDE EFFECTS

One of the key aspects of navigating cancer treatments is understanding the different treatment options available. These can include surgery, chemotherapy, radiation therapy, immunotherapy, targeted therapy, and hormone therapy, among others. Each treatment option has its own benefits and potential side effects, so it is essential to work closely with your healthcare team to determine the most suitable approach for your specific type and stage of cancer.

Navigating cancer treatments and managing side effects is a challenging yet essential aspect of the cancer journey, both for patients and their caregivers. From chemotherapy and radiation therapy to surgery and immunotherapy, the array of treatment options can be overwhelming, each with its own set of potential benefits and side effects. As a caregiver, supporting a loved one through this process requires patience, empathy, and a deep understanding of the physical and emotional toll that treatment can exact.

Chemotherapy, often considered the cornerstone of cancer treatment, can be particularly taxing on the body, leading to a range of side effects such as nausea, fatigue, hair loss, and weakened immune function.

As a caregiver, I have witnessed firsthand the toll that chemotherapy can take on my loved one's physical and emotional well-being. Supporting them through these challenging times involves providing practical assistance with daily tasks, such as meal preparation and transportation to medical appointments, as well as offering emotional support and encouragement to help them cope with the rigors of treatment.

Radiation therapy, another common cancer treatment, presents its own set of challenges and side effects, including skin irritation, fatigue, and changes in appetite. As a caregiver, I have learned to anticipate and address these side effects proactively, offering comfort measures such as gentle skincare, relaxation techniques, and nutritional support to help alleviate discomfort and promote healing. Additionally, providing emotional support and reassurance during radiation therapy sessions can help ease anxiety and boost morale during this challenging time.

Surgery, while often a necessary component of cancer treatment, can also be physically and emotionally demanding for patients and caregivers alike. As a caregiver, supporting a loved one through surgery involves not only providing practical assistance with pre-operative preparations and post-operative care but also offering emotional support and reassurance throughout the process. Helping my loved one cope with feelings of fear, uncertainty, and vulnerability surrounding surgery requires empathy, patience, and a willingness to listen and validate their concerns.

Immunotherapy, a newer approach to cancer treatment,

offers promising potential for some patients but can also come with its own set of side effects, including fatigue, flu-like symptoms, and autoimmune reactions. As a caregiver, staying informed about the latest advancements in cancer treatment and collaborating closely with healthcare providers to monitor and manage side effects is essential in ensuring the safety and well-being of my loved one undergoing immunotherapy.

Navigating cancer treatments and managing side effects is a journey fraught with challenges, but it is also a journey filled with hope, resilience, and the unwavering determination to overcome adversity. My role, as a caregiver, is to provide unwavering support and encouragement to my loved one as they navigate the difficulties of treatment, offering comfort, compassion, and companionship every step of the way. Together, we face the challenges of cancer treatment with courage, strength, and a steadfast belief in the power of love and support to overcome even the greatest of obstacles.

Managing side effects is another crucial aspect of cancer treatment. While the side effects can vary depending on the type of treatment, some common side effects include fatigue, nausea, hair loss, pain, and changes in appetite. It is important to communicate openly with your healthcare team about any side effects you may be experiencing, as they can provide guidance and support to help.

alleviate these symptoms. Additionally, there are various supportive care services available, such as nutrition counseling, pain management, and integrative therapies, which can help improve your overall well-being during treatment.

EMOTIONAL & PSYCHOLOGICAL SUPPORT: SHARING MY STRATEGIES FOR BEING THERE IN TIMES OF NEED

Being there for someone with cancer during their times of need is incredibly important. It can provide them with the support, comfort, and strength they need to navigate through their journey. Here are my strategies for being there for someone with cancer:

Active Listening: One of the most crucial strategies is to be an active listener. Give the person your undivided attention, allowing them to express their thoughts, fears, and emotions. Avoid interrupting or offering unsolicited advice. Instead, validate their feelings and provide a safe space for them to share.

Empathy and Compassion: Show empathy and compassion towards a person with cancer. Understand that they may be experiencing a wide range of emotions, including fear, anger, and sadness. Be patient and supportive, offering a shoulder to lean on and a listening ear whenever they need it.

Practical Support: Offer practical support to alleviate some of the burdens they may be facing. This can include helping with household chores, running errands, or providing transportation to medical appointments. By taking care of these tasks, you can allow them to focus on their treatment and well-being.

Emotional Support: Be a source of emotional support for the person with cancer. Offer words of encouragement, reassurance, and positivity. Let them know that you are there for them, no matter what. Engage in activities that bring them joy and provide a distraction from their illness.

Respect Boundaries: Respect the person's boundaries and preferences. Understand that they may need time alone or may not always want to talk about their illness. Be sensitive to their needs and give them space when necessary. Let them take the lead in determining how much support they require.

Educate Yourself: Take the time to educate yourself about their specific type of cancer and treatment options. This will allow you to have informed conversations and provide relevant support. It also shows that you care and are invested in their well-being.

Stay Positive and Hopeful: Maintain a positive and hopeful attitude when interacting with a person with cancer. Offer words of encouragement and remind them of their strength and resilience. Your positivity can be contagious and help them maintain a positive mindset throughout their journey.

Remember, everyone's experience with cancer is unique,

so it is important to adapt your strategies based on the individual's needs and preferences. By being there for someone with cancer in their times of need, you can make a significant difference in their journey towards healing and recovery.

CHAPTER III

Learning about Heart Conditions & Their Effects on Health

Throughout my personal journey of learning about heart conditions and their effects on health, I have gained a deep understanding of the impact these conditions can have on individuals. It all started when a close family member was diagnosed with a heart condition, which sparked my curiosity and desire to educate myself on the subject.

As I delved into the world of heart conditions, I was astounded by the complexity and intricacy of the human heart. I learned about various types of heart conditions, such as coronary artery disease, arrhythmias, and heart failure. Each condition presented its own set of challenges and potential consequences for the individual's overall health and well-being.

Witnessing the physical and emotional toll that heart conditions can take on individuals was truly eye-opening. It became clear to me that these conditions not only affect the heart itself but also have a profound impact on every aspect of a person's life. From daily activities to long-term plans, the presence of a heart condition can significantly alter one's lifestyle and perspective.

On top of that, it has been discovered that managing and treating heart conditions frequently calls for a multidisciplinary approach. A comprehensive care plan that is customized to each patient's unique needs is created through a collaborative effort involving cardiologists, nurses, dietitians, and other healthcare professionals. In addition to treating the patient's physical symptoms, this interdisciplinary approach also tries to take care of their psychological and emotional health.

Also learned about the importance of early detection and prevention strategies for heart conditions. Regular check-ups, maintaining a healthy lifestyle, and managing risk factors such as high blood pressure, cholesterol levels, and diabetes are crucial in reducing the likelihood of developing heart conditions. Education and awareness play a vital role in empowering individuals to take control of their heart health and make informed decisions.

I discovered the significance of support systems in coping with the effects of heart conditions. Whether it is the unwavering support of family and friends, or the guidance provided by support groups and online communities, having a strong network can make a world of difference. Sharing experiences, exchanging knowledge, and finding solace in the stories of others who have faced similar challenges can provide a sense of comfort and reassurance.

I have come to appreciate the resilience and strength of individuals living with heart conditions. Their determination to overcome obstacles, adapt to new circumstances, and maintain a positive outlook on life is truly inspiring. It serves as a reminder that even in the face of adversity, the human spirit has the capacity to thrive and find hope.

My personal journey of learning about heart conditions and their effects on health has been transformative. It has deepened my empathy and understanding for individuals facing these challenges and has motivated me to advocate for heart health awareness. By sharing my knowledge and experiences, I hope to contribute to a world where heart conditions are better understood, prevented, managed, and improving the overall well-being of individuals affected by these conditions.

WALKING ALONGSIDE THOSE WITH HEART CONDITIONS

Walking alongside those with heart conditions has been a journey that has deeply impacted me on both a personal and professional level. It is a journey that began with a sense of empathy and compassion, as I witnessed firsthand the challenges, fears, and uncertainties faced by individuals living with heart conditions and their loved ones. From the moment of diagnosis, I knew that I wanted to be there for them, offering support, encouragement, and a listening ear every step of the way.

As I walked alongside those with heart conditions, I quickly realized the importance of education and awareness. Many individuals and their families were overwhelmed by the complexity of their condition and the multitude of treatment options available. Therefore, I made it my mission to provide them with clear, understandable information about their diagnosis, treatment options, and lifestyle modifications. By empowering them with knowledge, I hoped to alleviate some of their anxiety and uncertainty, enabling them to make informed decisions about their care.

The journey that each person has with heart disease is distinct, so we must customize our approach to suit their requirements and preferences. Walking with people who have heart issues has also shown me how important it is to provide individualized care and support. I have grown adept at tailoring my support to each person's and their family's specific needs, whether that be through emotional support, help managing medication, or guidance through the healthcare system.

In addition to offering support to individuals with heart conditions, I have also been there for their caregivers and loved ones. Caring for someone with a heart condition can be emotionally and physically draining, and caregivers often need support and respite themselves. By offering a compassionate ear, practical assistance, and encouragement, I have sought to ease their burden and provide them with the support they need to navigate their caregiving journey with strength and resilience.

I have learned how crucial it is to promote optimism and hope from walking beside people who have heart issues. People who suffer from chronic illnesses may experience overwhelming feelings of hopelessness and despair. Because of this, I have made it my mission to instill optimism and hope in the people I support, telling them that their circumstances do not define who they are and that there are always good reasons to keep fighting and working toward a better tomorrow.

I have walked alongside those with heart conditions as they have faced the ups and downs of their treatment journey. From the highs of successful surgeries and improvements in their symptoms to the lows of setbacks and complications. Through it all, I have remained a constant source of encouragement and reassurance, reminding them that they are never alone in their journey.

In addition to providing emotional support, I have also advocated for those with heart conditions within the healthcare system. Whether it is ensuring that they receive timely and appropriate care, advocating for their rights and preferences, or addressing gaps in the healthcare system that impact their access to care, I have been a vocal advocate for their needs and concerns. By amplifying their voices and championing their rights, I have sought to ensure that they receive the high-quality, patient-centered care they deserve.

Dealing with those that have heart conditions has taught me the importance of resilience and perseverance. Despite facing numerous challenges and setbacks, individuals living with heart conditions have shown incredible strength and courage in their journey. Their resilience has inspired me to remain steadfast in my support, even in the face of adversity, and to continue advocating for better care and support for all individuals living with heart disease.

Those individuals with heart conditions have deepened my appreciation for the fragility and preciousness of life. Witnessing the resilience and strength of individuals facing serious health challenges has reminded me to cherish each moment and live life to the fullest. It is a lesson that I carry with me every day as I continue to support and advocate for those living with heart conditions.

In conclusion, walking alongside those with heart

conditions has been a journey of empathy, compassion, and growth. It is a journey that has taught me the importance of education, personalized care, advocacy, and resilience. Most importantly, it is a journey that has reaffirmed my commitment to being there for others, offering support, encouragement, and hope as they navigate the challenges of living with heart disease.

SUPPORTING LIFESTYLE CHANGES & MANAGEMENT STRATEGIES

Supporting lifestyle changes and management strategies for heart conditions is essential in promoting the well-being and longevity of individuals affected by cardiovascular disease. As a caregiver, I recognize the importance of assisting my loved one in adopting healthy lifestyle habits and adhering to recommended management strategies to reduce the risk of complications and improve overall heart health.

One crucial aspect of supporting lifestyle changes for heart conditions is promoting a heart-healthy diet. This involves encouraging my loved one to consume a balanced diet rich in fruits, vegetables, whole grains, lean proteins, and healthy fats while limiting their intake of processed foods, saturated fats, sodium, and added sugars. By providing guidance on meal planning, grocery shopping, and cooking heart-healthy meals, I can help my loved one make informed dietary choices that support their cardiovascular health.

Regular physical activity is another key component of managing heart conditions, and as a caregiver, I play a vital role in encouraging and facilitating exercise. This may involve assisting my loved one in finding enjoyable and appropriate forms of physical activity, such as walking, swimming, or cycling, and incorporating exercise into their daily routine. Additionally, I provide encouragement, support, and companionship during exercise sessions to help motivate my loved one to stay active and committed to their fitness goals.

Managing stress is also crucial for heart health, and as a caregiver, I help my loved one develop effective stress management strategies. This may include practicing relaxation techniques such as deep breathing, meditation, or yoga, as well as engaging in enjoyable hobbies and activities that promote relaxation and well-being. By encouraging my loved one to prioritize self-care and find healthy outlets for managing stress, I can help reduce their risk of stress-related cardiovascular complications.

Ensuring medication adherence is another essential aspect of supporting management strategies for heart conditions. As a caregiver, I help my loved one stay organized with their medications, including keeping track of dosages, refill schedules, and potential side effects. Additionally, I encourage open communication with healthcare providers regarding any concerns or questions about medications, and I advocate for my loved one's needs and preferences to ensure they receive the best possible care.

Creating a supportive and heart-healthy environment at home is also critical for managing heart conditions. This involves promoting a smoke-free environment, encouraging adequate sleep, and minimizing exposure to environmental pollutants and toxins that can exacerbate cardiovascular health issues. Additionally, I assist my loved one in maintaining regular follow-up appointments with healthcare providers, monitoring their blood pressure, cholesterol levels, and other relevant health markers to track their progress and adjust treatment as needed.

Education is a powerful tool in supporting lifestyle changes and management strategies for heart conditions. As a caregiver, I provide my loved ones with accurate and up-to-date information about their condition, treatment options, and risk factors, empowering them to make informed decisions about their health. By helping them understand the importance of adhering to recommended lifestyle changes and management strategies, I can motivate and empower my loved one to take an active role in managing their heart health and reducing their risk of cardiovascular complications.

Supporting lifestyle changes and management strategies for heart conditions is a multifaceted endeavor that requires collaboration, commitment, and compassion. As a caregiver, I am dedicated to assisting my loved one in adopting healthy lifestyle habits, adhering to recommended management strategies, and prioritizing their cardiovascular health. By providing guidance, encouragement, and support, I strive to empower my loved one to take control of their heart health and live a full and active life despite their condition.

JOURNEYING THROUGH MEDICAL PROCEDURES & SURGERIES: MY INSIGHTS AND TIPS

Going through medical procedures and surgeries can be a daunting and overwhelming experience. As someone who has personally gone through these challenges, I understand the importance of having insights and tips to navigate through this journey. Here are my personal insights and tips for getting through medical procedures and surgeries:

Educate Yourself: Take the time to research and understand the procedure or surgery you will be undergoing. This will help alleviate any fears or uncertainties you may have and allow you to ask informed questions to your healthcare provider.

Communicate with Your Healthcare Team: Open and honest communication with your healthcare team is crucial. Make sure to voice any concerns or questions you may have before, during, and after the procedure or surgery. They are there to support you and provide the necessary information.

Follow Pre-Procedure Instructions: It is important to follow any pre-procedure instructions given by your healthcare team. This may include fasting, medication adjustments, or specific preparations. Adhering to these instructions will help ensure a smooth procedure.

Have a Support System: Surround yourself with a strong support system of family and friends who can provide emotional support during this time. They can accompany you to appointments, offer a listening ear, and help with practical matters.

Prepare for Recovery: Before the procedure or surgery, make sure to prepare your home for a comfortable recovery. Stock up on necessary supplies, arrange for transportation if needed, and create a relaxing environment to aid in your recovery.

Manage Pain and Discomfort: Follow your healthcare provider's instructions for managing pain and discomfort after the procedure or surgery. This may include taking prescribed medications, using ice packs, or practicing relaxation techniques.

Take Care of Yourself: During the recovery period, prioritize self-care. This includes getting enough rest, eating nutritious meals, staying hydrated, and engaging in gentle physical activity as recommended by your healthcare provider.

Seek Emotional Support: It is normal to experience a range of emotions during the recovery process. If you find yourself feeling overwhelmed, anxious, or depressed, do not hesitate to seek professional help or join support groups where you can connect with others who have gone through similar experiences.

Remember, everyone's experience with medical procedures and surgeries is unique, and it is important to listen to your body and advocate for your needs. By following these insights and tips, I hope you can navigate through this journey with confidence and resilience.

PROVIDING EMOTIONAL SUPPORT FOR PATIENTS & FAMILIES ON THE HEART HEALTH JOURNEY

Providing emotional support for a family member on their heart health journey is crucial in helping them navigate through the challenges they may face. It is a role that requires empathy, understanding, and patience. Here are nine paragraphs outlining strategies and tips for providing emotional support during this journey:

Be a good listener: One of the most important ways to provide emotional support is by being a good listener. Allow your family members to express their fears, concerns, and emotions without judgment. Give them your full attention and validate their feelings.

Inform yourself: Take the time to learn about heart conditions and their effects on health. This will not only help you understand what your family members are going through, but it will also enable you to provide them with accurate information and support.

Offer reassurance: It is common for individuals with heart conditions to experience anxiety and fear. Offer reassurance by reminding your family members that they are not alone on this journey. Let them know that you are there to support them every step of the way.

Encourage healthy habits: Promote a healthy lifestyle by encouraging your family members to adopt heart-healthy habits. This can include regular exercise, a balanced diet, and stress management techniques. Offer to join them in these activities to provide additional support and motivation.

Attend medical appointments together: Accompany your family members to their medical appointments. This shows your support and allows you to stay informed about their condition and treatment plan. Take notes during the appointments to help them remember valuable information.

Be patient and understanding: Understand that your family members may experience physical and emotional difficulties throughout their heart health journey. Be patient and understanding during these times, offering them a safe space to express their emotions without judgment.

Help with practical tasks: Offer to help with practical tasks such as meal preparation, house chores, or transportation to medical appointments. These small gestures can alleviate some of the stress and burden your family member may be experiencing.

Encourage self-care: Remind your family members to prioritize self-care. Encourage them to engage in activities they enjoy, practice relaxation techniques, and seek support from other sources such as support groups or counseling if needed.

Celebrate milestones: Celebrate milestones and achievements along the way. Whether it is reaching a specific health goal or completing a successful medical procedure, acknowledge and celebrate these accomplishments to boost your family member's morale and motivation.

Remember to provide emotional support is an ongoing process. Be there for your family members consistently and adapt your support as their needs change. Your presence and understanding can make a significant difference in their heart health journey.

CHAPTER IV.

Embracing the Challenges of Mental Illness

Throughout my personal journey of embracing the challenges of mental illness, I have come to understand the profound impact it can have on every aspect of my life. It is a constant battle that requires resilience, self-compassion, and a support system that understands and accepts me for who I am. While it can be overwhelming at times, I have learned to find strength in my struggles and use them as opportunities for growth and self-discovery.

One of the most important aspects of embracing mental illness is acknowledging and accepting my emotions. It is crucial to allow myself to feel and express my emotions without judgment or shame. By doing so, I am able to process and understand my feelings, which leads to a greater sense of self-awareness and emotional well-being.

Another key component of embracing mental illness is practicing self-care. This involves prioritizing my physical, emotional, and mental well-being. Whether it is engaging in activities that bring me joy, practicing mindfulness and meditation, or seeking professional help when needed, self-care plays a vital role in managing my mental health.

Building a dedicated support system has been instrumental

in my journey. Surrounding myself with understanding and compassionate individuals who validate my experiences and provide a safe space for me to express myself has been invaluable. Whether it is through therapy, support groups, or close friends and family, having a support system that I can rely on has made a significant difference in my ability to navigate the challenges of mental illness.

Embracing the challenges of mental illness has taught me the importance of setting boundaries. It is crucial to recognize my limits and communicate them effectively to others. By doing so, I can protect my mental health and ensure that I am prioritizing my well-being.

In addition, education and advocacy have played a significant role in my journey. By educating myself about mental health conditions and advocating for greater understanding and acceptance, I can break down the stigma surrounding mental illness and promote a more inclusive and supportive society.

While gaining an understanding of the difficulties posed by mental illness has helped me realize the value of not. I have learned to get back up and keep going forward despite obstacles and setbacks. Learned about my inner strength and capacity for overcoming hardship because of these difficulties.

It takes a profoundly personal and transforming journey

to accept the challenges of mental illness. Setting limits, being educated, advocating for oneself, accepting oneself, self-care, a solid support network, and resilience are all necessary. I have developed personally because of accepting these difficulties, and I now know how to navigate the difficulties of mental health bravely and gracefully.

MY UNDERSTANDING OF DIFFERENT MENTAL HEALTH CONDITIONS & THEIR IMPACT

Throughout my personal journey of understanding the different mental health conditions and their impact, I have gained a profound insight into the complexities of these conditions and the challenges they present. It is crucial to recognize that mental health is not a one-size-fits-all concept, and there are various conditions that can affect individuals in unique ways.

One of the most common mental health conditions is anxiety. As someone who has experienced anxiety firsthand, I know how overwhelming and debilitating it can be. It is characterized by excessive worry, fear, and a constant feeling of unease. Anxiety can significantly impact a person's daily life, making it difficult to concentrate, sleep, and engage in social activities.

Depression is another mental health condition that I have encountered on my journey. It is more than just feeling sad or down; it is a persistent feeling of hopelessness, loss of interest in activities, and a lack of energy. Depression can make even the simplest tasks seem overwhelming, and it can have a profound impact on one's overall well-being.

Bipolar disorder is a mental health condition that involves

extreme mood swings, ranging from manic episodes of high energy and euphoria to depressive episodes of sadness and low motivation. Living with bipolar disorder can be challenging as it requires managing these intense mood shifts and finding stability in everyday life.

Post-traumatic stress disorder (PTSD) is a mental health condition that can develop after experiencing or witnessing a traumatic event. It can cause intrusive thoughts, nightmares, and intense emotional and physical reactions. Understanding the impact of PTSD is crucial in providing support and empathy to those who have gone through traumatic experiences.

Eating disorders, such as anorexia nervosa and bulimia nervosa, are mental health conditions that affect a person's relationship with food and body image. These conditions can have severe physical and psychological consequences, and they require a comprehensive approach to treatment and support.

Attention-deficit/hyperactivity disorder (ADHD) is a neurodevelopmental disorder that affects both children and adults. It is characterized by difficulties with attention, hyperactivity, and impulsivity. Understanding the impact of ADHD can help individuals and their loved ones navigate the challenges and find effective strategies for managing symptoms.

Schizophrenia is a complex mental health condition that

involves a range of symptoms, including hallucinations, delusions, and disorganized thinking. It can significantly impact a person's perception of reality and their ability to function in daily life. Understanding the challenges faced by individuals with schizophrenia is crucial in providing appropriate support and treatment.

My personal journey of understanding the different mental health conditions and their impact has taught me the importance of empathy, compassion, and education. Each condition is unique, and it is essential to approach mental health with an open mind and a willingness to learn. By understanding these conditions, we can create a more supportive and inclusive society for individuals facing mental health challenges.

BREAKING DOWN STIGMA: MY EXPERIENCE SUPPORTING LOVED ONES FACING MENTAL ILLNESS

During my own experience of helping family members with mental illness, I have witnessed the profound impact it can have on their lives and the lives of those around them. It is a journey filled with both challenges and moments of growth, requiring patience, understanding, and unwavering support. Here are seven paragraphs outlining my experience and the lessons I have learned along the way.

When I first learned that a loved one was facing mental illness, I was filled with a mix of emotions - concern, fear, and uncertainty. However, I quickly realized that it was essential to educate myself about their condition and the numerous ways it could manifest. This knowledge helped me better understand their struggles and offer the right kind of support.

One of the most important lessons I have learned is the power of empathy. Mental illness can be an isolating experience and knowing that someone utterly understands and empathizes with their struggles can make a world of difference. I made it a point to actively listen to my loved ones, validate their feelings, and let them know that they are not alone.

Supporting a loved one with mental illness also means being their advocate. Accompanied them to therapy sessions, doctor appointments, and support groups, ensuring that they receive the necessary care and treatment. Being their advocate has empowered them to navigate the complex healthcare system and find the resources they need.

Patience is another crucial aspect of supporting loved ones facing mental illness. Recovery is not linear, and there may be setbacks along the way. It is important to be patient and understanding, allowing them to progress at their own pace. Celebrating even the smallest victories and offering reassurance during challenging times can make a significant impact.

Self-care is often overlooked when supporting loved ones with mental illness, but it is vital. I have learned that I cannot pour from an empty cup, and taking care of my own mental and emotional well-being is essential. Engaging in activities that bring me joy, seeking support from friends and professionals, and setting boundaries have helped me maintain my own mental health.

Communication plays a crucial role in supporting loved ones facing mental illness. Found that open and honest conversations about their condition, treatment options, and their needs have fostered a sense of trust and understanding. Regular check-ins and asking how they are truly feeling have helped me gauge their well-being and offer appropriate support.

Supporting loved ones with mental illness requires a network of support. I have reached out to support groups, online communities, and mental health professionals to gain insights and guidance. Building a support system not only benefits my loved one but also provides me with the resources and encouragement I need to continue supporting them effectively.

My experience of supporting loved ones facing mental illness has taught me the importance of empathy, patience, self-care, and effective communication. It is a journey that requires continuous learning, adaptability, and unwavering support. By being there for our loved ones, we can make a positive difference in their lives and help them navigate the challenges of mental illness.

EXPLORING TREATMENT OPTIONS:

THERAPY, MEDICTION, AND SUPPORT GROUPS

When it comes to treating mental health patients, there are various options available that can help individuals on their journey towards recovery and well-being. Three common treatment options include therapy, medication, and support groups. Each of these approaches plays a unique role in addressing mental health conditions and providing the necessary support for patients.

Therapy: Therapy, also known as counseling or psychotherapy, is a widely used treatment option for mental health patients. It involves meeting with a trained therapist who provides a safe and confidential space for individuals to explore their thoughts, emotions, and behaviors. Therapists utilize various techniques and approaches such as cognitive-behavioral therapy (CBT), dialectical behavior therapy (DBT), and psychodynamic therapy to help patients gain insight, develop coping skills, and make positive changes in their lives.

Medication: Medication can be an essential component of treatment for individuals with mental health conditions. Psychiatrists and other healthcare professionals may prescribe medications such as antidepressants, antianxiety drugs, mood stabilizers, or antipsychotics to help manage symptoms. These medications work by balancing brain chemicals and can be effective in reducing symptoms such as depression, anxiety, or mood swings. It is important to note that medication should always be prescribed and monitored by a qualified healthcare professional.

Support Groups: Support groups provide a valuable source of emotional support and understanding for individuals facing mental health challenges. These groups bring together individuals who share similar experiences or conditions, allowing them to connect, share their stories, and offer support to one another. Support groups can be facilitated by mental health professionals or run by peers who have personal experience with mental health conditions. They provide a safe space for individuals to express themselves, learn from others, and gain a sense of belonging and community.

Self-Help Strategies: In addition to professional treatment options, individuals can also benefit from incorporating self-help strategies into their mental health journey. These strategies may include practicing mindfulness and relaxation techniques, engaging in regular physical exercise, maintaining a healthy lifestyle, and seeking out resources such as self-help books or online forums. Self-help strategies empower individuals to take an active role in their own well-being and can complement other treatment approaches.

Holistic Approaches: Some individuals may find holistic approaches beneficial in their mental health treatment. These approaches focus on the interconnectedness of the mind, body, and spirit and may include practices such as yoga, meditation, acupuncture, or herbal remedies. It is important to consult with healthcare professionals before incorporating any alternative or complementary treatments to ensure their safety and effectiveness.

Hospitalization: In severe cases where individuals are at risk of harming themselves or others, hospitalization may be necessary. Psychiatric hospitals provide a structured and supportive environment where individuals can receive intensive treatment and monitoring. Hospitalization aims to stabilize individuals in crisis and ensure their safety until they can transition to less intensive levels of care.

Integrated Treatment: Integrated treatment involves a comprehensive approach that combines different treatment modalities to address the unique needs of individuals with mental health conditions. This approach may involve a combination of therapy, medication, support groups, and other interventions tailored to the individual's specific needs. Integrated treatment recognizes that mental health conditions are complex and require a comprehensive approach that considers the biological, psychological, and social factors influencing an individual's well-being.

It is important to remember that the most effective treatment plan for mental health patients may vary depending on the individual and their specific needs. A personalized approach, in collaboration with healthcare professionals, can help individuals find the right combination of treatments that work best for them.

CHAPTER V

Supporting Physical and Mental Well-being

Supporting the physical and mental well-being of family members with mental health challenges is a multifaceted endeavor that requires empathy, understanding, and initiative-taking care. As a caregiver, I recognize the importance of addressing both the physical and emotional aspects of my family member's health to promote overall well-being and resilience.

One crucial aspect of supporting physical and mental well-being is prioritizing a healthy lifestyle. Encouraging regular exercise, nutritious eating habits, adequate sleep, and stress management techniques can help maintain physical health while also supporting mental health. By incorporating these healthy habits into our daily routine as a family, we promote a sense of well-being and vitality that contributes to resilience and overall quality of life.

Open communication and emotional support are essential for fostering a supportive environment where my family member feels understood, accepted, and valued. By actively listening to their concerns, validating their experiences, and offering empathy and encouragement, I create a safe space for them to express themselves and seek support when needed. This open and supportive dynamic strengthens our bond as a family and promotes resilience in the face of mental health challenges.

Access to appropriate mental health care and treatment is critical for supporting the well-being of family members with mental health conditions. I work closely with healthcare providers to ensure my family members receive comprehensive and compassionate care that addresses their unique needs and preferences. This may involve therapy, medication management, support groups, and other evidence-based treatments that promote recovery and well-being.

Encouraging meaningful social connections and activities is another important aspect of supporting the well-being of family members with mental health challenges. Whether it is participating in hobbies, spending time with friends and loved ones, or engaging in community activities, fostering a sense of belonging and connection can help alleviate feelings of isolation and loneliness and promote mental and emotional well-being.

Self-care is equally important for both my family members and me as a caregiver. By prioritizing my own well-being and modeling healthy self-care practices, I demonstrate the importance of self-care and resilience in managing mental health challenges. This may involve setting boundaries, seeking support from friends and family, engaging in activities that bring joy and relaxation, and practicing mindfulness and stress management techniques.

Education and advocacy play a crucial role in supporting the well-being of family members with mental health challenges. I actively seek out information and resources to better understand their condition and treatment options, empowering myself to advocate for their needs and preferences effectively. By raising awareness and challenging stigma surrounding mental health, I work to create a more supportive and inclusive environment for my family members and others facing similar challenges.

Finally, fostering hope, resilience, and a sense of purpose is essential for supporting the well-being of family members with mental health challenges. By emphasizing their strengths, acknowledging their progress, and celebrating their achievements, I instill confidence and optimism in their ability to overcome obstacles and thrive despite their condition. Together, we navigate the ups and downs of mental health challenges with courage, resilience, and unwavering support, knowing that we are stronger together as a family.

HOLISTIC APPROACHES
TO MENTAL ILLNESS

Holistic approaches to mental illness focus on treating the whole person rather than just the symptoms of the condition. These approaches recognize that mental health is influenced by several factors, including physical, emotional, social, and spiritual well-being. By addressing these several aspects, holistic approaches aim to promote overall wellness and improve mental health outcomes. Here are seven paragraphs exploring different holistic approaches to mental illness.

Mindfulness and Meditation: Mindfulness and meditation practices are integral components of holistic approaches to mental illness. These practices involve focusing one's attention on the present moment and cultivating a non-judgmental awareness of thoughts, feelings, and sensations. By practicing mindfulness and meditation, individuals can develop skills to manage stress, reduce anxiety, and enhance overall mental well-being.

Exercise and Physical Activity: Physical activity plays a crucial role in holistic approaches to mental illness. Engaging in regular exercise releases endorphins, which are natural mood-boosting chemicals in the brain. Exercise also helps reduce symptoms of depression and anxiety, improves sleep quality, and enhances self-esteem. Incorporating physical activity into one's routine can contribute to improved mental health and overall well-being.

Nutrition and Diet: A healthy diet is essential for maintaining optimal mental health. Certain nutrients, such as omega-3 fatty acids, B vitamins, and magnesium, have been found to support brain function and improve mood. Holistic approaches to mental illness emphasize the importance of a balanced diet that includes fruits, vegetables, whole grains, lean proteins, and healthy fats to support overall mental well-being.

Social Support and Connection: Building and maintaining strong social connections is vital for mental health. Holistic approaches to mental illness emphasize the importance of social support networks, such as family, friends, and support groups. These connections provide emotional support, reduce feelings of isolation, and promote a sense of belonging, all of which are crucial for overall mental well-being.

Creative Expression and Art Therapy: Engaging in creative activities, such as art therapy, can be therapeutic for individuals with mental illness. Art therapy allows individuals to express their thoughts, emotions, and experiences through various art forms, such as painting, drawing, or writing. This form of self-expression can help individuals process and cope with their emotions, reduce stress, and promote self-discovery and personal growth.

Alternative Therapies: Holistic approaches to mental illness often incorporate alternative therapies, such as acupuncture, yoga, and aromatherapy. These therapies aim to restore balance and promote overall well-being by addressing the body, mind, and spirit. Alternative therapies can help individuals manage symptoms of mental illness, reduce stress, and improve overall quality of life.

Self-Care and Stress Management: Self-care practices are essential for maintaining mental health and well-being. Holistic approaches to mental illness emphasize the importance of self-care activities, such as getting enough sleep, practicing relaxation techniques, setting boundaries, and engaging in activities that bring joy and fulfillment. By prioritizing self-care and stress management, individuals can better cope with the challenges of mental illness and promote their overall mental well-being.

Holistic approaches to mental illness recognize the interconnectedness of various aspects of a person's life and aim to promote overall wellness. By incorporating practices such as mindfulness, exercise, nutrition, social support, creative expression, alternative therapies, and self-care, individuals can enhance their mental health and well-being. These approaches provide a comprehensive and integrative approach to mental illness that considers the whole person, leading to improved mental health outcomes and a better quality of life.

MY PERSONAL INSIGHTS ON NUTRITION, EXERCISE, AND SLEEP FOR OVERALL HEALTH

I have learned a lot about the connections between sleep, exercise, and nutrition in promoting overall wellness as I make my way towards optimum health and well-being. Incorporated these elements into my daily routine because I understand how important they are to leading a healthy, active lifestyle.

Nutrition serves as the foundation of my approach to health, as I have come to understand the profound impact of food choices on both physical and mental well-being. Embracing a diet rich in whole, nutrient-dense foods such as fruits, vegetables, lean proteins, and whole grains, I prioritize nourishing my body with the essential vitamins, minerals, and antioxidants it needs to thrive.

By focusing on real, unprocessed foods and minimizing consumption of refined sugars, unhealthy fats, and processed foods, I support my body's natural ability to function optimally and maintain a strong immune system.

Regular exercise is another cornerstone of my health routine, as I have experienced firsthand the transformative effects of physical activity on both body and mind. Incorporating a variety of activities such as strength training, cardiovascular exercise, yoga, and outdoor activities, I have found joy and fulfillment in moving my body and challenging myself to new heights. Exercise not only helps me maintain a healthy weight and improve physical fitness but also boosts mood, reduces stress, and enhances cognitive function, contributing to a sense of vitality and well-being.

Sleep plays a critical role in supporting overall health and vitality, and I have learned to prioritize rest and relaxation as essential components of my wellness routine. Recognizing the restorative power of sleep, I strive to create a sleep-friendly environment and establish consistent bedtime routines that promote relaxation and restful sleep. By prioritizing quality sleep and aiming for seven to eight hours of rest each night, I support my body's natural rhythms and optimize its ability to repair and regenerate, ensuring I wake up feeling refreshed and energized each morning.

Mindful eating practices have become integral to my approach to nutrition, as I have cultivated a deeper awareness of my body's hunger and satiety cues and learned to savor and enjoy my meals mindfully. By slowing down and paying attention to the sensory experience of eating, I have developed a greater appreciation for the flavors, textures, and aromas of food, fostering a more positive and satisfying relationship with eating. Mindful eating not only helps me make healthier food choices but also promotes digestion, reduces stress, and enhances overall well-being.

Incorporating regular movement and physical activity into my daily life has become second nature, as I have embraced the joy and benefits of staying active. Whether it is taking brisk walks in nature, practicing yoga in the comfort of my home, or engaging in fun recreational activities with friends and family, I find ways to move my body that brings me joy and fulfillment. By making exercise a priority and finding activities that I enjoy, I stay motivated and committed to maintaining an active lifestyle that supports my overall health and well-being.

Creating a relaxing bedtime routine has become an essential part of my self-care practice, as I have discovered the power of winding down and preparing my body and mind for restful sleep. Whether it is taking a warm bath, practicing gentle stretching or meditation, or reading a book before bed, I prioritize activities that promote relaxation and signal to my body that it is time to unwind. By establishing a consistent bedtime routine and creating a calming sleep environment, I set the stage for restful and rejuvenating sleep that supports my overall health and well-being.

Practicing gratitude and mindfulness has enriched my approach to nutrition, exercise, and sleep, as I have learned to cultivate a deeper sense of awareness and appreciation for the present moment. By savoring the simple pleasures of nourishing food, invigorating movement, and restful sleep, I enhance my overall sense of well-being and fulfillment. Mindfulness also helps me make conscious choices that support my health and vitality, empowering me to live with intention and purpose.

Seeking support and accountability from loved ones and community resources has been instrumental in my journey towards optimal health and well-being. By surrounding myself with like-minded individuals who share similar health goals and values, I gain inspiration, motivation, and encouragement to stay committed to my wellness journey. Whether it is joining a fitness class, participating in a cooking club, or connecting with online communities, I find strength and support in the shared experiences and camaraderie of others on similar paths.

My personal insights on nutrition, exercise, and sleep have shaped my approach to overall health and well-being, empowering me to make informed choices that support my physical, mental, and emotional vitality. By prioritizing nourishing foods, regular movement, restful sleep, and mindful living, I cultivate a lifestyle that fosters balance, resilience, and a profound sense of well-being.

EMBRACING MINDFULNESS AND STRESS REDUCTION TECHNIQUES FOR PATIENTS AS A CAREGIVERS

Throughout my personal experience as a caregiver, I have learned the importance of stress reduction techniques in maintaining overall well-being. Dealing with the challenges of illness can be overwhelming, but implementing effective strategies can make a significant difference. The following nine strategies for patients and caregivers to reduce stress:

Mindfulness and Meditation: Practicing mindfulness and meditation can help calm the mind and reduce stress. Taking a few minutes each day to focus on the present moment can provide a sense of peace and clarity.

Deep Breathing Exercises: Deep breathing exercises are a simple yet powerful way to relax the body and mind. By taking slow, deep breaths and focusing on the breath, you can activate the body's relaxation response and reduce stress.

Physical Activity: Engaging in regular physical activity, such as walking, yoga, or swimming, can help release endorphins and reduce stress levels. It also promotes overall well-being and improves mood.

Time Management: Effective time management can help reduce stress by allowing patients and caregivers to prioritize tasks and allocate time for self-care. Creating a schedule and setting realistic goals can provide a sense of control and reduce feelings of overwhelm.

Social Support: Connecting with others who are going through similar experiences can provide emotional support and reduce stress. Joining support groups or seeking counseling can be beneficial for both patients and caregivers.

Relaxation Techniques: Incorporating relaxation techniques, such as progressive muscle relaxation or guided imagery, into daily routines can help reduce stress and promote relaxation.

Self-Care: Taking time for self-care is essential for both patients and caregivers. Engaging in activities that bring joy and relaxation, such as reading, listening to music, or taking a bath, can help reduce stress and improve overall well-being.

Healthy Lifestyle Choices: Making healthy lifestyle choices, such as eating a balanced diet, getting enough sleep, and limiting alcohol and caffeine intake, can support stress reduction. These choices provide the body with the necessary resources to cope with stress.

Seeking Professional Help: If stress becomes overwhelming or persistent, it is important to seek professional help. Mental health professionals can provide guidance and support in developing effective stress management strategies.

Both patients and caregivers can better manage the difficulties of illness and preserve their wellbeing by putting these stress-reduction strategies into practice. Never forget how important it is to put self-care first and ask for help when you need it.

CHAPTER VI

Nurturing Caregivers and Practicing Self-Compassion

As a caregiver, I have come to understand the importance of nurturing myself and practicing self-compassion as essential components of maintaining my own well-being while caring for others. Through my experiences, I have learned that caregiving can be both rewarding and challenging, and that prioritizing my own needs is not only necessary but also beneficial for those I care for.

Nurturing caregivers involves recognizing and honoring the physical, emotional, and spiritual needs of oneself. This may include setting boundaries to protect personal time and energy, seeking support from friends and family, and engaging in activities that bring joy and relaxation. By prioritizing self-care and nurturing my own well-being, I am better equipped to show up fully for my loved ones, offering them the support and care they need.

Practicing self-compassion is an essential aspect of caregiving, as it allows me to offer myself the same kindness and understanding that I extend to others. By acknowledging my own limitations and imperfections with gentleness and acceptance, I cultivate a sense of inner peace and resilience that enables me to navigate the challenges of caregiving with greater grace and compassion. Self-compassion also helps me maintain a healthy perspective, recognizing that I am doing the best I can in a challenging situation and that it is okay to ask for help when needed.

One way I nurture myself as a caregiver is by prioritizing activities that replenish my energy and bring me joy. Whether it is taking a walk-in nature, practicing yoga, reading a book, or spending time with loved ones, I carve out time in my schedule for activities that nourish my soul and replenish my spirit. By honoring my own needs and engaging in activities that bring me fulfillment, I ensure that I have the energy and resilience to continue caring for others with compassion and grace.

Another crucial component of nurturing caregivers is asking for help from others. Whether it is joining a support group for caregivers, confiding in a trusted friend, or seeking guidance from a therapist, reaching out for support can provide a sense of validation, understanding, and connection that alleviates feelings of isolation and burnout. By sharing my experiences and receiving support from others, I cultivate a sense of community and solidarity that strengthens my resilience and empowers me to continue caring for my loved ones with compassion and grace.

Being kind and understanding to oneself, particularly in times of struggle or self-doubt, is an important part of practicing self-compassion. Instead of criticizing myself for perceived shortcomings or mistakes, I offer myself words of encouragement and reassurance, recognizing that I am doing the best I can in a challenging situation. By cultivating self-compassion, I develop a sense of inner resilience and self-worth that enables me to navigate the difficulties of caregiving with greater ease and grace.

Setting boundaries is an important aspect of nurturing caregivers, as it allows me to protect my own well-being and prevent burnout. This may involve saying no to additional responsibilities, delegating tasks to others, or taking breaks when needed to rest and recharge. By honoring my own needs and limitations, I ensure that I have the energy and resilience to continue caring for my loved ones with compassion and grace.

Practicing gratitude is another powerful way to nurture caregivers and cultivate a sense of well-being. By focusing on the blessings and positive aspects of my life, I shift my perspective from scarcity to abundance, fostering a sense of joy and appreciation that uplifts my spirits and sustains me through challenging times. Whether it is keeping a gratitude journal, expressing thanks to others, or simply pausing to savor life's small moments of beauty and grace, practicing gratitude reminds me of the abundance of love and blessings that surround me each day.

Taking care of my physical health is an important aspect of nurturing caregivers and practicing self-compassion. This may involve eating a balanced diet, getting regular exercise, and prioritizing sleep and relaxation. By nourishing my body with healthy food, movement, and rest, I support my overall well-being and build resilience to stress and illness, ensuring that I have the energy and vitality to continue caring for my loved ones with compassion and grace.

Nurturing caregivers and practicing self-compassion are essential aspects of maintaining well-being and resilience while caring for others. By prioritizing self-care, seeking support from others, setting boundaries, practicing gratitude, and taking care of my physical health, I cultivate a sense of inner strength and resilience that enables me to navigate the challenges of caregiving with compassion, grace, and resilience.

RECOGNIZING THE UNIQUE CHALLENGES FACED BY CAREGIVERS

Throughout my personal journey as a caregiver, I have faced numerous unique challenges that have tested my strength and resilience. Being a caregiver is a role that comes with immense responsibility and can often be emotionally and physically demanding. Here are nine paragraphs outlining the unique challenges faced by caregivers:

One of the most significant challenges I have encountered as a caregiver is the constant juggling of multiple responsibilities. Balancing the needs of the person I am caring for with my own personal and professional obligations can be overwhelming at times. It requires careful planning, organization, and the ability to prioritize effectively.

Another challenge I have faced is the emotional toll that caregiving can take. Witnessing a loved one's decline in health or experiencing their pain and suffering can be heartbreaking. It is essential to find healthy coping mechanisms and seek support from others who understand the challenges of caregiving.

The physical demands of caregiving can also be challenging. Assisting with daily activities such as bathing, dressing, and feeding may require physical strength and endurance. It is crucial to take care of my own physical well-being to ensure that I can continue to provide the best care possible.

Financial strain is another significant challenge faced by caregivers. Medical expenses, home modifications, and other costs associated with caregiving can quickly add up. Navigating the complex healthcare system and finding resources to alleviate the financial burden can be daunting.

Social isolation is a common challenge for caregivers. The demands of caregiving can often limit social interactions and leisure activities. It is important to try to maintain connections with friends and family and seek out support groups or online communities for caregivers.

Dealing with the uncertainty of a loved one's health condition can be mentally and emotionally exhausting. Not knowing what the future holds or how the person I am caring for will progress can create anxiety and stress. Finding healthy ways to cope with uncertainty, such as practicing mindfulness or seeking therapy, is crucial.

Advocating for the person I am caring for can be a significant challenge. Navigating the healthcare system, communicating with doctors, and ensuring that their needs are met requires assertiveness and persistence. It is essential to educate myself about their condition and be their voice when necessary.

Caregiver burnout is a real and prevalent challenge. The constant demands of caregiving can leave caregivers feeling physically and emotionally drained. It is crucial to prioritize self-care, set boundaries, and seek respite care to prevent burnout and maintain my own well-being.

The grief and loss experienced by caregivers can be profound. As a caregiver, I may witness the decline of a loved one's health or eventually face their passing. Processing these emotions and finding ways to cope with grief is an ongoing challenge.

Being a caregiver presents unique challenges that require strength, resilience, and a support system. It is essential to prioritize self-care, seek support from others, and educate oneself about the resources available. Despite the challenges, caregiving can also be a rewarding and meaningful experience, allowing for deep connections and personal growth.

BUILDING A SUPPORT NETWORK: MY ADVICE FOR CAREGIVERS

One of the most important things I have done as a caregiver to keep my wellbeing while giving care has been to establish a support system.

When I first started on this journey, I felt overwhelmed and isolated, but I quickly realized that I could not do it all alone. I needed a community around me, people who understood the challenges and could offer practical help and emotional support.

I began by reaching out to close family members and friends, explaining the situation and the kind of help I needed. It was heartwarming to see how many were willing to lend a hand, whether it was running errands, cooking a meal, or just being there to listen. This immediate circle became the core of my support network, providing a safety net on days when the burden felt too heavy to carry alone.

Beyond my personal connections, I sought out local caregiver support groups. Meeting others in similar situations gave me a sense of camaraderie and belonging. We shared tips, resources, and sometimes just the comfort of knowing we were not alone in our struggles. These groups often had knowledgeable speakers who provided insights into caregiving strategies and self-care, which proved invaluable.

Online communities and forums also became a part of my extended support system. They were accessible at any hour, which was particularly helpful during late-night moments of worry or stress. Connecting with caregivers from around the world broadened my perspective and introduced me to diverse ways of coping and caring.

I did not neglect professional support either. Consulting with healthcare professionals, counselors, and social workers helped me navigate the complex healthcare system and address the emotional toll caregiving can take. Their expert advice on managing specific health conditions and mental health support was a lifeline during the most challenging times.

Volunteer services and non-profit organizations offered additional layers of support. From respite care to home modifications and transportation services, these resources helped lighten the load. They allowed me to take much-needed breaks and focus on my own health without feeling guilty or worried about the level of care my loved one was receiving.

I also made it a point to educate myself. I attended workshops and read extensively on caregiving topics. Knowledge empowered me to make informed decisions and advocate effectively for my loved one's needs. It also helped me communicate better with medical professionals and service providers.

To keep my support network strong, I learned the importance of reciprocity. While I often leaned on others, I also offered my support when I could. Sharing my experiences, lending an ear, or helping another caregiver in a small way fostered a sense of community and purpose that went beyond my individual role.

I found strength in self-reflection and mindfulness practices. Taking time for introspection helped me understand my limits and recognize when to ask for help. Mindfulness kept me grounded and prevented burnout, ensuring that I could continue to provide the best care possible while maintaining my own health and happiness. Building this support network was not just about finding help; it was about creating a community of care that surrounded both my loved one and me.

CHAPTER VII.

Effective Communication and Advocacy

As a caregiver, I have come to understand that effective communication is not just about conveying information; it is about connecting with others on a level that fosters understanding and empathy. When I began this role, I quickly learned that being able to articulate my loved one's needs, as well as my own, was essential in ensuring the best care and support.

Advocacy became a significant part of my daily routine. It meant standing up for my loved one's rights and making sure their voice was heard, especially in medical settings where they might feel vulnerable or overlooked. I had to be assertive yet respectful, asking questions and seeking clarifications to make informed decisions together with healthcare providers.

I also realized the importance of active listening. Sometimes, my loved ones struggled to express their concerns or desires, and it was crucial for me to listen carefully, read between the lines, and validate their feelings. This built trust and made them feel valued, which in turn made it easier to discuss and plan their care.

Clear and consistent communication with other family members was equally important. Organized regular family meetings to discuss updates, changes in health status, and to delegate tasks. This helped prevent misunderstandings and ensured that everyone was on the same page regarding our loved one's care.

Documentation played a key role in effective communication. Kept detailed records of medical appointments, treatments, and daily care activities. These notes were invaluable during doctor's visits and when coordinating with other caregivers, ensuring continuity of care, and preventing any details from slipping through the cracks.

In advocating for my loved one, I also had to navigate the complexities of insurance and healthcare systems. Educated myself on policies and procedures to effectively communicate our needs and rights. This often-involved lengthy discussions with insurance representatives and healthcare administrators to secure the services and coverage necessary for quality care.

I found that maintaining open lines of communication with professional caregivers was vital. By sharing insights into my loved one's preferences and routines, I helped create a more personalized and comfortable care experience. Regular check-ins with these professionals allowed us to address any issues promptly and collaboratively.

Sometimes, despite my best efforts, conflicts arose. In such situations, I focused on problem-solving and negotiation techniques. Approached each issue with the intent to understand the other party's perspective and find a mutually acceptable solution, always keeping my loved one's best interests at heart.

I learned to advocate for myself as a caregiver. I communicated my limits and sought support when needed, recognizing that caring for myself was not selfish but necessary. By doing so, I could continue to provide the best possible care for my loved one without sacrificing my own well-being. Effective communication and advocacy have been challenging but rewarding aspects of caregiving, and they have taught me skills that extend far beyond this role.

MY INSIGHTS INTO COMMUNICATING EFFECTIVELY WITH PATIENTS AND CAREGIVERS

As a caregiver, I have learned that communicating effectively with patients is an art that requires patience, empathy, and clarity. From the moment I began caring for individuals with various needs, I recognized that each patient has their unique way of understanding and processing information, and it is my job to adapt to that.

One of the first things I do when establishing communication with a new patient is to get to know them personally. I ask about their interests, background, and preferences. This not only helps build rapport but also gives me insight into how to approach conversations about their care.

I make it a point to always speak to my patients with respect and dignity, regardless of their cognitive or physical abilities. I never talk down to them or use baby talk; instead, I maintain a conversational tone that acknowledges their adulthood and individuality.

Active listening is another critical component of effective communication. When my patients speak, I give them my full attention, making eye contact and nodding to show that I am engaged. I listen not just to their words but also to their tone and body language, which can convey much more than speech alone.

I strive to ensure that my explanations are clear and straightforward when discussing medical terms or care plans. I avoid jargon and break down complex concepts into understandable language. If I sense any confusion, I rephrase my explanation or use analogies that relate to their experiences.

When it comes to sensitive topics or difficult news, I choose my words carefully and provide the information in a compassionate manner. I allow space for patients to express their emotions and ask questions, and I offer comfort and reassurance as needed.

I also recognize the importance of nonverbal communication. A gentle touch on the shoulder, a warm smile, or a reassuring nod can all convey care and compassion without saying a word. These gestures often speak volumes to patients who may be feeling vulnerable or scared.

Feedback is essential in ensuring that my communication methods are effective. I regularly check in with my patients to see if they understand the information I have provided and if they have any concerns. This two-way dialogue helps me refine my approach and tailor my communication to better meet their needs.

I document key conversations and decisions made with my patients. This practice not only helps maintain continuity of care but also serves as a reference for future discussions. It ensures that both the patient and I have a clear understanding of the care plan and any changes that may occur over time. Communicating effectively with patients is a cornerstone of caregiving, and it is a skill that I continuously work to improve.

STANDING UP FOR PATIENTS'
NEEDS AND RIGHTS

As a caregiver, I have come to realize that standing up for my patients' needs and rights is not just a responsibility—it is a calling. From the very beginning, I understood that my role was to be more than just a provider of care; I needed to be an advocate, a voice for those who might struggle to speak up for themselves.

I remember the first time I had to assertively communicate with a healthcare professional on behalf of a patient. It was daunting, but the clear necessity to ensure my patient received the appropriate level of care gave me the courage to speak out. That experience taught me the importance of being well-informed about my patients' conditions and their rights as individuals.

In every interaction with doctors, nurses, and other healthcare providers, I make it a point to clearly articulate my patients' needs. I do not shy away from asking questions or requesting further explanations when something is not clear or does not seem right. My patients depend on me to understand the nuances of their care and to ensure that their treatment plans are followed correctly.

I have also learned the significance of informed consent. I

take the time to explain procedures and treatments to my patients in a way they can understand, ensuring they are fully aware of their options and the potential outcomes. It is crucial that they feel empowered to make decisions about their own health and well-being.

There have been times when I have encountered resistance or bureaucracy that hindered my patients' access to necessary services or treatments. In these moments, I have had to be tenacious, utilizing every resource at my disposal —whether it is through persistent phone calls, written appeals, or reaching out to patient advocacy groups—to break down barriers.

Privacy and confidentiality are rights I guard zealously. I am meticulous about protecting my patients' personal health information, understanding that trust is a fundamental component of the caregiver-patient relationship. I advocate for their privacy in all settings, ensuring that their sensitive information is shared only with those who need to know for the sake of their care.

I also stand up for my patients' right to dignity and respect. This means honoring their cultural, spiritual, and personal values in all aspects of their care. I strive to create an environment where they feel safe and respected, free from any form of discrimination or judgment.

When it comes to end-of-life care, advocating for my patients' wishes is especially poignant. I work closely with them and their families to ensure that advance directives and living wills are established and honored, so that their preferences for care are respected during the most vulnerable times.

Education is a powerful tool in advocacy. I continually educate myself on the latest healthcare policies, patient rights legislation, and best practices in caregiving. This knowledge equips me to better navigate the healthcare system and to challenge any injustices or lapses in care that my patients may face.

I recognize that self-care is essential to being an effective advocate. I must be at my best—physically, mentally, and emotionally—to stand up for my patients effectively. By taking care of myself, I ensure that I can continue to fight for my patients' needs and rights with the energy and dedication they deserve. Advocacy is not just part of my job; it is a commitment I have made to each person I care for, and it is one I uphold with honor and integrity.

EMPOWERING PATIENTS AND CAREGIVERS TO MAKE INFORMED DECISIONS

Empowering patients and caregivers to make informed decisions is crucial in providing quality healthcare. As a healthcare professional, I understand the importance of ensuring that patients and caregivers have the knowledge and tools they need to make decisions that are in their best interest. By empowering them to be active participants in their own healthcare, we can improve outcomes and enhance the overall patient experience.

One way to empower patients and caregivers is through education. Providing them with information about their medical condition, treatment options, and potential risks and benefits allows them to make informed decisions about their care. This education should be tailored to their individual needs and preferences, and presented in a clear and accessible manner so that they can fully understand their options.

Another important aspect of empowering patients and caregivers involves them in the decision-making process. This means listening to their concerns, answering their questions, and taking their preferences into account when developing a treatment plan. By actively involving them in the decision-making process, we can ensure that their values and goals are reflected in their care, leading to more satisfying outcomes for all parties involved.

It is also important to provide patients and caregivers with the necessary support to make informed decisions. This includes discussing the potential benefits and risks of various treatment options, as well as providing resources for further information and support. By offering this guidance and support, we can help patients and caregivers navigate the complexities of the healthcare system and make decisions that align with their values and preferences.

Additionally, empowering patients and caregivers to make informed decisions involves promoting shared decision-making between healthcare providers and patients. This collaborative approach allows patients and caregivers to actively participate in the decision-making process, ensuring that their voices are heard, and their concerns are addressed. By fostering this partnership, we can enhance patient satisfaction and improve health outcomes.

Furthermore, empowering patients and caregivers to make informed decisions requires fostering a culture of transparency and trust within the healthcare system. By being honest and open with patients and caregivers about their condition, treatment options, and potential outcomes, we can build trust and confidence in the healthcare provider-patient relationship. This transparency helps patients and caregivers feel more empowered to make decisions about their care and engage in their treatment plan.

Another important aspect of empowering patients and caregivers is ensuring that they have access to all the information they need to make informed decisions. This includes providing information about their medical condition, treatment options, and potential outcomes, as well as discussing any uncertainties or risks associated with each option. By providing this information in a clear and accessible manner, we can help patients and caregivers make decisions that align with their values and preferences.

Honoring patients' and caregivers' autonomy and decision-making skills is essential to enabling them to make educated choices. Recognizing that patients and caregivers have the authority to make decisions about their care that are in their best interests is crucial. They are the experts on their own lives and experiences. With patients and caregivers, we can establish a solid and trustworthy relationship by honoring their autonomy and allowing them to participate in the decision-making process.

In addition, empowering patients and caregivers to make informed decisions means acknowledging the unique challenges and barriers they may face in the healthcare system. This includes considering factors such as cultural beliefs, socioeconomic status, and limited access to resources. By recognizing these challenges and working to address them, we can better support patients and caregivers in making decisions that are right for them.

Furthermore, empowering patients and caregivers to make

informed decisions involves providing them with the necessary tools and resources to navigate the healthcare system. This includes helping them understand their rights as patients, navigate the complexities of insurance coverage, and access support services such as counseling or peer support groups. By providing these resources, we can help patients and caregivers feel more confident in making decisions about their care.

Encouraging patients and caregivers to ask questions and seek clarification when necessary is another way to empower them to make informed decisions. Fostering transparent communication and establishing a secure environment for discussion can assist patients and caregivers in feeling more at ease in standing up for themselves and their loved ones. We can empower individuals to make decisions that are consistent with their values and preferences by promoting initiative-taking caregiving.

Empowering patients and caregivers to make informed decisions is essential in providing patient-centered care. By educating them, involving them in the decision-making process, providing support, fostering transparency and trust, respecting their autonomy, acknowledging their unique challenges, and providing resources, we can empower patients and caregivers to make decisions that are in their best interest. As a healthcare professional, I am committed to supporting patients and caregivers in making informed decisions and advocating for their needs in the healthcare system.

CHAPTER VIII

Reflecting on My Journey as a Compassionate Caregiver

My journey caring for family members as a caregiver has been a deeply personal and transformative experience, shaping my understanding of love, resilience, and the true meaning of family. It began unexpectedly, with the realization that my loved one needed assistance due to age, illness, or disability. Initially, I felt a mix of emotions—compassion, responsibility, and a tinge of apprehension—but I knew deep down that I was ready to take on the role of caregiver out of love and duty.

As I embarked on this journey, I quickly realized that being a caregiver meant more than just providing physical assistance; it meant being a source of emotional support, companionship, and advocacy for my family members. From helping with daily tasks like bathing and dressing to offering a listening ear and a shoulder to lean on during tough times, I learned to be there for my loved one in every possible way.

One of the most profound aspects of my journey as a caregiver has been witnessing the resilience and strength of my family member in the face of adversity. Despite the challenges they faced, whether it be managing a chronic illness, recovering from surgery, or adapting to life with a disability, they approached each day with courage and grace, inspiring me to do the same.

Moreover, caring for a family member has taught me the importance of patience and empathy. There are moments of frustration and exhaustion, to be sure, but I have learned to approach each situation with kindness and understanding. By putting myself in my loved one's shoes and seeing the world through their eyes, I have gained a deeper appreciation for their struggles and triumphs.

In addition, my journey as a caregiver has highlighted the importance of self-care. It is easy to become so focused on the needs of my family member that I neglect my own well-being, but I have learned that taking care of myself is essential for providing the best possible care. Whether it is finding time for relaxation and hobbies or seeking support from friends and family, prioritizing self-care has helped me maintain my physical and emotional health throughout this journey.

My role as a caregiver has strengthened my bond with my family members in profound ways. Through the difficulties, we have forged a connection built on love, trust, and mutual respect. Our shared experiences have deepened our understanding of each other and brought us closer together, strengthening the fabric of our family in the process.

Aside from the psychological aspects of caregiving, I have also had to deal with the day-to-day difficulties of organizing medical attention, managing prescription drugs, and standing up for my family members in the medical system. Making sure my loved one gets the best care possible has become my responsibility, and I have taken on everything from making doctor's appointments to looking into treatment options and interacting with healthcare professionals.

The necessity of creating a support system has been brought to light by my experience as a caregiver. I have discovered that I do not have to go through this journey alone, and I can get assistance from other caregivers, go to support groups, hire professional caregivers, or use respite care services. Through asking for help when I need it, I have been able to share the load of taking care of others and find comfort in the fact that I am not alone.

Had to face my own limitations and fears because of my work as a caregiver. Wondered if I am capable of handling the responsibilities involved in providing care at times when I have felt doubtful and uneasy. Every new obstacle I have encountered has led me to uncover a previously unknown source of inner strength and fortitude.

My journey caring for family members as a caregiver has been a profound testament to the power of love, compassion, and human connection. While it has not always been easy, it has been a journey filled with moments of joy, growth, and deep meaning. Through it all, I remain committed to being there for my family members, providing them with the care, support, and dignity they deserve.

RESOURCES FOR FURTHER
SUPPORT AND INFORMATION

There are numerous resources available for support and information regarding mental health, heart disease, and dementia. Support groups, hotlines, and online forums provide a sense of community for individuals facing these challenges. Websites like www.wellmentally.org, the National Institute of Mental Health, American Heart Association, and Alzheimer's Association offer valuable information on symptoms, treatments, and coping strategies. Seeking professional help from therapists, cardiologists, or neurologists is also crucial for managing these conditions effectively.

Encouraging continued support and advocacy for individuals facing health challenges is a cause close to my heart, driven by a deep sense of compassion and a belief in the inherent worth and dignity of every individual. Throughout my journey, I have witnessed firsthand the profound impact that ongoing support and advocacy can have on those navigating health challenges, empowering them to overcome obstacles and live their fullest lives.

In addition to fostering support and advocacy on a broader scale, I have also provided individualized support to those facing health challenges in my personal life. Whether it is offering a listening ear, providing practical assistance, or accompanying them to medical appointments, I have sought to be a source of support and encouragement for those navigating challenging times.

Caregivers believe it is their duty to stand up for their patients' rights and needs. Learned early on that being an advocate is part of my job, starting with the first time I had to speak firmly to a healthcare worker for a patient. I always make sure to communicate clearly about what my patients need and ask questions if things are not clear.

Explain medical procedures to my patients so they can make informed choices and fight for their access to needed services. Keep their personal health information private because trust is key in caregiving. Respect their dignity and cultural values and ensure their end-of-life wishes are known and followed.

To do this well, I keep learning about healthcare policies and patient rights. I also take care of myself to stay strong for my patients. Advocacy is not just part of my job; it is a promise I keep with honor and integrity.

NAVIGATING THE HEALTHCARE SYSTEM: PRACTICAL TIPS AND RESOURCES

Understand Your Insurance: Familiarize yourself with your health insurance coverage. Know the extent of your benefits, including copays, deductibles, and out-of-pocket expenses.

Choose the Right Provider: Select healthcare providers who are in-network to maximize your coverage. Research their qualifications and reputation to ensure quality care.

Ask Questions: Do not hesitate to ask your healthcare provider questions about your diagnosis, treatment options, and any concerns you may have. Understanding your healthcare plan is crucial for informed decision-making.

Keep Records: Maintain a file with all your medical records, test results, and prescriptions. This will help you track your health history and share information with new providers.

Stay Informed: Stay up to date on healthcare news, advancements, and changes in policies. Being informed empowers you to make better decisions about your health.

Utilize Preventive Care: Take advantage of preventive

services like vaccinations, screenings, and check-ups. Early detection can often lead to more effective treatment.

Seek Second Opinions: If facing a significant medical decision, do not hesitate to seek a second opinion. Different perspectives can provide clarity and peace of mind.

Explore Telehealth Options: Telehealth services offer convenient access to healthcare professionals through virtual appointments. Consider this option for non-emergency consultations.

Advocate for Yourself: Be an active participant in your healthcare. Voice your concerns, preferences, and goals to ensure your needs are met.

Stay Organized: Keep a calendar with your appointments, medications, and follow-ups. Being organized helps you stay on top of your healthcare regimen.

Financial Assistance Programs: Explore financial assistance programs offered by hospitals, pharmaceutical companies, and government agencies. These programs can help alleviate the financial burden of healthcare costs.

Community Resources: Tap into community resources like support groups, health fairs, and wellness programs. These resources can provide valuable information and emotional support.

Patient Advocacy Organizations: Connect with You Belong @ www.WellMentally.com/resources